"SEA MOSS, THE AMAZING SEAWEED"
"The 92 Vitamin & Mineral Multivitamin."

By T.C. Browdy

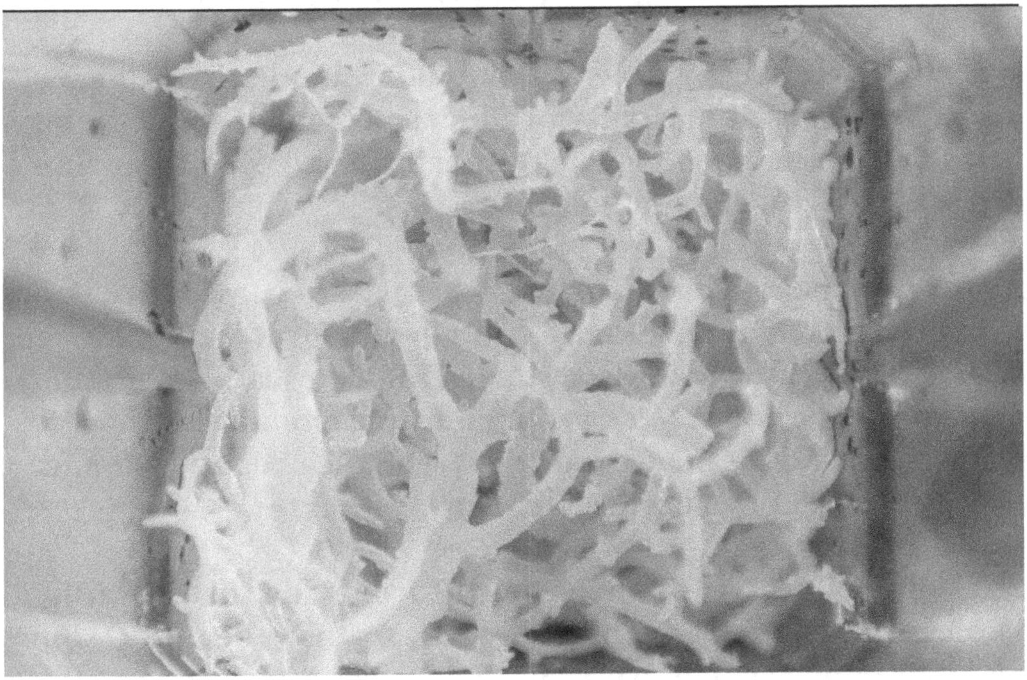

I was always taught that "there's nothing new under the sun."

Scientists estimate the Ocean aka the Sea has been in existence in excess of over 3 billion years. Yes, that long. Before mankind was here, there was the ocean. Some people even believe that all mankind, animals and beings come from the ocean. I am not the Creator, so I have no opinion in that regard.

But Sea Moss, can be dated back 14,000 years and the Chinese using it as early as 600 B.C. and the British using it as a source of nutrition in 400 B.C. Back many years ago it was used to cure infections and congestion issues in humans and animals.

It is now used for its carrageenan to boost immunity, enhance beauty and is used in beauty products, personal products and helps to control blood pressure, infertility and even treat skin diseases like eczema and hair loss.

My partner being from Jamaica, wherein Sea Moss is drank on a daily basis, taught me many years back how to make this red sea algae or sea weed and we started making sea moss gel and opened a store and started selling massive amounts to those wanting to combat the Coronavirus, enhance beauty, enhance energy and heal from other ailments or diseases.

So if you're ready to discover the gift from God that is waiting to bless you with energy, body healing, fertility, beautiful skin and hair and even help with fighting cancer cells, keep reading and you will understand the greatness of this Superfood and why I want to share it with every human being under the sun

CONTENTS

INTRODUCTION

During the pandemic that took us all by storm, we all began looking and searching for alternative methods to not only survive but to also help boost our immune system and get rid of any potential threats that could be associated with the virus symptoms that even resembled or showed a sign of getting Covid-19 or Coronavirus.

If you've been around, you've probably been hearing of one way that has become extremely popular to help combat, build the immune system and fight Covid-19, flu, cold and even pneumonia symptoms is something called Seamoss. Seamoss is a very unique looking, seaweed plant derived from the Ocean that is called by many different names, namely; Irish Sea Moss, Sea Moss, Irish Moss, Chondrus Crispus, Genus Gracilaria.

There aren't only many different names, but thousands of different species. The question remains and I've been asked by many customers and family members is, "Are all of these aliases in and of one another or is there a difference?" Alias, new thing, immune booster, Covid-19 cure, flu and cold saviour? Well, if you've been hearing about the Sea Moss trend as some call it, then you have probably heard it being one or the other or all.

Whether it's a big deal to you or no big deal, if you want to add it into your diet or just take it now and then or maybe you just don't know exactly how to Google this product or even know which one is the correct one… Hmmm….

Maybe you just want to try it and don't know how to actually implement it into recipes or make it yourself. Regardless of your reasoning for inquiring about Sea Moss or your interest in probing further into this astounding, God given gem, you have chosen the right book and the right start because this after all is a new phenomenon and a great adventure to improving your overall health, skin, hair, mindset, diet, nutrition and overall body.

So what exactly is this pasta looking substance that everyone is raving about? Why is it called Irish Sea Moss and is it found in Caribbean waters, European waters? What are the benefits? Is it really true to its word? Does it really work? Did Dr. Sebi really survive on sea moss alone? Questions, questions, questions….
Answers, answers, answers….

Irish Sea Moss, Irish Moss, Corpus Crispus, Genus Gracilaria or Sea Moss, people Google and search for different names and in this book we will be telling you the origin, differences, definitions, uses, benefits, mineral and vitamin content and much much more….

So, mostly anybody and everybody that is on the internet, watches YouTube, listens to or have read about Nipsey Hussle, read or heard about Dr. Sebi, listened to Lisa (left eye) Lopez, buy from Etsy and/or Amazon. If you have listened to any of these people or buy on any of these platforms, you have undoubtedly heard of Irish Sea Moss, Sea Moss, Irish Moss, Corpus Crispus, Genus Gracilaria and if you haven't heard about it in depth, you have undoubtedly, at least heard the word, words or names and didn't know what it was and what it does for you or maybe you heard what it can do, but just wasn't quite sure how to consume it or how to implement it into your diet. This is the reason why I have decided to write this book. I would like to inform the public of this phenomenon, amazing herb and benefits if I may.

In this book I will inform you of my introduction into the Sea Moss World, its benefits, best way to consume it and why everybody needs this nutrient-rich, high mineral food in their daily diet along with testaments from people that have taken this food for many different reasons and have achieved great success from cold and flu-like symptoms, skin disorders to mineral deficiency to energy production and on and on and on…..

Before we get started, I would like to take the opportunity at this time to thank you so much for purchasing my book. I am very appreciative of all of my customers on every level from my sea moss store to my books and I am so grateful for so much positive energy, love and support, since beginning my sea moss business in February of 2020.

Now, let's get started……..

CHAPTER ONE
"DR. SEBI"

Our Dear, Blessed, Beloved Dr. Sebi……. Peace and love to you, our great ancestor….

I have come to the understanding in life that there are people in this world that came here that are just different, atypical, distinct. They are here for a reason. They come to bless us. They come to help us look at things in a different light. They're angels in human form. So many of us have come across these people, sometimes one has come and sometimes many have come. Either way, I can attest to the fact that they can come for a reason, a season or a lifetime. Our beloved Dr. Sebi has come and he has come for a lifetime, if only we take our time and listen to his videos, his book, products and understand his legacy.

Through sound and the internet we have been blessed with a spirit, a being, a voice that will be with us and among us as long as we allow him to be with us and within us. This angel in human form may be with us for the rest of our life if we allow it or he may just be with us for the time period in which we choose to listen to him or search for him and for that time period only. Life is about choices. You choose in which manner you want him in your life, you make the decision, but please choose wisely.

Many years ago, 18, maybe 20 years to be more precise, I would speak to my uncle on a daily basis, sometimes twice a day. Our conversations would mostly consist of religion, health, exercise, our family, life. I recall him first asking me, "Have you heard of Dr. Sebi? I said, "No. I don't know who that is. Who is that?" He goes, "Really Tiya? You don't know who Dr. Sebi is?" The guy who went to the Supreme Court with 70 witnesses and proved that an alkaline diet can cure AIDS, HIV, herpes, diabetes, cancer, mental illness, etc.…."

"Really? I don't believe that." If that was the case I would have heard about him by now," I responded nonchalantly.

"No, you wouldn't."How would you know if you don't look for it? It's not something that's talked about, so you won't know anything about it unless you see these videos" (cd's back then or tapes.) "Oh, okay," I say to myself.

To make a long story short, the conversation did continue and after him making a huge deal out of me not knowing who Dr. Sebi was I started looking into who this mysterious person was that very few people knew anything about...

I am not going to stay on Dr. Sebi too long but due to my research into his logic on herbal medicine, specifically Sea Moss, there were a few things that stood out to me as I started to do some research on him.

One thing that stood out for me, is when our beloved Dr. Sebi told his mother, I have cured 13 AIDS patients and she said, "They're going to get you."

I ask is this true? Lisa (left eye) Lopez, dead in a car crash, whom he treated.
Michael Jackson, whom he was know for treating, gone….
Nipsey Hussle, gone…

If he's not a threat to the world, the pharmaceutical companies, doctors, hospitals, the system then why is he along with many other famous people, gone? Just asking a question and I think a great question to ask.

This man was amazing regarding his holistic approach to healing the human body and I really do not feel that he gets the credit that he deserves.

I could actually go on and on about the accomplishments of Dr. Sebi, the people that he's cured (without formal education), the mucous that he's eliminated in the body and alkalined the body from an acidic nature by eating certain foods. But, I will save that for the next book.   For right now, we'll get back to Sea Moss.

As I stated previously, the reason why I even began to understand, research and inform people and eventually get a store to sell this superfood is all due to me educating myself about the benefits of this great, highly nutritious food and the journey began with Dr. Sebi and a Jamaican grandmother (now deceased, that I didn't know was Jamaican originally) and my partner, whom is also Caribbean. If you all are in anyway familiar with Dr. Sebi, you will know that he fasted regularly and would fast with only eating sea moss for 40 and sometimes 60 days and this was very intriguing for me. My partner's family and my grandmother's family consumed this drink regularly and so have I along the way of this long road of having kids and post-partum and even utilizing and making into a baby formula.

One of the questions of fact that has arisen quite often is, can you actually go for a long period of time with eating Sea Moss alone and still get your daily vitamins and minerals? This and many other questions will be answered in the next chapters...

CHAPTER TWO
"ORIGIN AND FACTS"

Irish Sea Moss or Jamaican Sea Moss; Same? Different? Hmmmm...

Now, that I have given you all a brief background as to the reasoning of me writing, selling and being totally enthralled with Sea Moss, I will now go more in depth as to what Irish Sea Moss actually is, cultivation and the differences between the two most popular sea mosses; Chondrus Crispus and Genus Gracilaria.

The Scientific name of Irish Sea Moss is Chondrus Crispus. It is a species of red algae and grows in the colder, more rocky parts of the Atlantic Coastlines of Europe and North America including the U.S. and Canada and particularly Ireland, when fresh it is soft and cartilaginous, meaning it is made of cartilage and varies in color from a greenish-yellow, through red, to dark purple or purplish-brown.

The principal constituent is mucilaginous or having a gelatinous consistency body form, in a more simpler term and made of polysaccharide carrageenan, which constitutes 55% of its dry weight. The organism also consists of nearly 10% of dry weight protein and about 15% dry weight mineral matter and very high in iodine, which produces thyroid hormones that is essential for the body, (which the body doesn't self-produce) and sulfur which builds and fixes DNA and protects cells from damage from disease and which also assists the body to metabolize food and contributes to skin, tendons and ligaments.

It is a seaweed with flat fan like leaves. Once placed into water you will see how the texture changes by becoming larger and then lightens up in color and emanates a sea-like odor and once placed into water and/or boiling water it forms a jelly like texture and will grow 20 to 100 times its size…

Chondrus Crispus aka Irish Sea Moss can be found in the ocean; from the ocean floor on a rock, from the middle intertidal zone, into the subtidal zone and can survive with minimal sunlight…. Irish Sea Moss's name originally became popular when there was a potato famine in Ireland in the 1800s. At the time people were starving and desperate for food and began eating the red algae off of the rocks due to food scarcity and due to millions of people dying from malnourishment related diseases. It allowed many people at the time to survive because of the high mineral and vitamin content.

Genus Gracilaria aka Jamaican Sea Moss and I must infer that Dr. Sebi did refer to this particular Sea Moss as Chondrus Crispus as being one in the same, but after much research I would like to inform you that there are slight differences in the two. Yes, there is. I am quite sure that many people was wondering about this question
because I was, so I took the time out and did the research myself, so just to reiterate, one is Chondrus Crispus aka Irish Sea Moss and one is Genus Gracilaria aka Jamaican Sea Moss or just Sea Moss and the structure is different and grown in different regions, both are high in mineral, Iodine and sulfur and great for the body.

I will note, that there are thousands of different species of sea mosses but the most talked about are the Irish Sea Moss (Chondrus Crispus) and Sea Moss or Jamaican Sea Moss(Genus Gracilaria).

Genus gracilaria is grown in warm climates, most notably around Jamaica and St. Lucia. It is found in warm waters throughout the world. Genus Gracilaria is not tolerable to temperatures below 10 degrees C (50 fahrenheit) and are found in all oceans except the Arctic Ocean including South America, Africa and Oceania. It is traditionally cultivated in the Western Pacific and as a source of agar.

Genus gracilaria, like its cousin Chondrus Crispus is also a red algae (Rhodophyta) and is a thicker and sticks more like seaweed. It has a wide range of tolerance for changing environmental conditions, like its cousin, when fresh it also is soft and cartilaginous and varies in color from a greenish-yellow, to a dark purple or purplish-brown. It, also like its cousin is high in iodine and sulfur and once placed into water and boiling water it will expand 20 to 100 times its size and will also emanate a sea-like odor.

Genus gracilaria is used as a food in not only Caribbean nations such as Jamaica and St. Lucia but also in Filipino, Hawaii, Japanese and Korean cuisines. Although, it is called a different name. It is termed ogonori ogo in Japan, gulaman in the Phlippines and used as a gelatin and in Jamaica it is known as Irish Moss and in Korea, kkosiraegi. Variations of the Genus Gracilaria is cultivated among Asia, South America, Africa and Oceania but is also found in the ocean on estuaries or bays, often in intertidal or shallow subtidal areas, less than one meter deep and can be attached to rocks or free floating.

Now, as I have given descriptions of these two sea mosses and some of the similarities, let's now compare the two:

Chondrus Crispus (Irish Sea Moss) vs. Genus Gracilaria (Sea Moss aka Jamaican Sea Moss)

#1. As stated earlier, Chondrus Crispus aka Irish Sea Moss is grown off of the Atlantic Coastlines and North American including the U.S. and Canada and in particular Ireland it's cousin Genus Gracilaria aka Jamaican Sea Moss is grown in a more warmer climate including Jamaica, St. Lucia, Asia, South America and Africa and is less leafy.

#2. Sea Moss is very accessible, abundant and plentiful while Irish Sea Moss is very scarce and really hard to come by. Irish Sea Moss is really hard to get from a vendor and more than likely if you are Googling Irish Sea Moss you are actually getting results for Sea Moss, Irish Moss aka Genus Gracilaria..

#3. Irish Sea Moss has a natural producing Carrageenan that gets extracted from the plant and is mostly utilized in dairy products as a thickening agent. That carrageenan found in Irish Sea Moss has been linked to inflammation, bloating and even food allergies, although there is a very small linkage to those side effects.

A similarity to note for the record between the two sea mosses is the presence of Anthocyanin which is found in cabbage, eggplant and blueberries and can contribute to the prevention of cancer and help improve one's memory.

#4. Irish Sea Moss (if you can find) and Sea Moss both have 92 out of the 102 trace minerals that the body is made from and is a vitamin/mineral powerhouse, so to speak.

Some of the 92 trace minerals that these two cousins carry is Iodine, sulfur, beta-carotene, Vitamins A, B, C, D, E and K, magnesium, manganese, calcium, phosphorus, zinc, potassium iodide, potassium bromide, selenium, natural silica, iron, B-complex, Folate, Copper, Sodium, Boron, Soluble potash, Phosphoric Acid, Carbohydrates including; Alginic Acid, Mannitol, Laminarin, Nitrogen and so many many more….

#5. As stated previously, it is quite rare to even find Irish Sea Moss that is actually from Ireland from a vendor and the price is much steeper than it's cousin, Sea Moss or Jamaican Sea Moss. The price per pound for Organic Irish Sea Moss will have a price tag of around $90.00 to $150.00 per pound and it's cousin, the Jamaican Sea Moss will run you around $35.00 to $100.00 per pound, depending on the supply and demand.

But, I will state that you cannot put a price tag on your health and the amount that you pay per pound if thinking in a logical, entrepreneurial sense it makes for a great business investment because although you are spending $50.00 to $100.00 per pound for the Sea Moss after soaking it in water the sea moss will reshape into 20 to 100 times its size and you can sell as a gel, so I do recommend buying raw and learning the dynamics of creating the gels and jarring it up and selling in your own online store. That is my advice from a business aspect.

Those are the main similarities and differences of the Sea Mosses.

In the next chapter we will be covering how to clean, prepare and consume Sea Moss gel.

CHAPTER 3
"Let's Get to Business!"

Now, as stated previously many times, the Irish Sea Moss is relatively difficult to purchase and if you actually do find a vendor it will be quite a bit more expensive. I personally do not see the necessity of buying the Irish Sea Moss due to the fact that both sea mosses contain the 92 minerals that we are looking for to attain optimal health and get the nutrients that we are seeking, so we sell and use Wild Crafted Sea Moss from Jamaica or St. Lucia.

Step One: The very first step that you must do is find a vendor or find someone that you would like to purchase your Sea Moss from.

Being a business owner, I purchase my Wild Crafted Sea Moss in bulk. My vendor is from Jamaica and he sells Jamaican Sea Moss and St. Lucia Sea Moss in bulk. He actually is my business partner's cousin and owns several restaurants in Miami and we actually travel to Miami to purchase the Sea Moss to make sure that we are getting a top of the line, high quality product. Now, just to explain a little, when I say top of the line. I am actually going to the facility and seeing where it is coming from and making sure it's genuine Sea Moss and not too sandy or too dirty because usually if it's too difficult clean due to too much sand it's usually not genuine. Because we have been doing this for so long, we can look at the sea moss and know fake versus real.

For your information, I do encourage anyone buying Sea Moss, especially for health and business purposes to get to understand real from fake because there are a lot of sea mosses that look authentic but are not and are pool grown or farm grown and will not provide the minerals and vitamins that the authentic sea moss provides.

I will provide ways to tell the difference at the end of this chapter.

But for right now let's get back to the steps of Sea Moss preparation.

I have purchased Sea Moss that was a bit more sandy and thinner and not as dried out and actually did not get as much gel when blended. I have had customers to tell me that the dried out Sea Moss that I also sell was fake and they just did not like the Jamaican Sea Moss versus St. Lucia Sea Moss. I will state that this particular Sea Moss was much cheaper but it did take much more to make just one jar of gel and many of my customers did not like the texture, so I made the business decision to pay much more and get a better texture with less product.

With the more thinner, sandier, cheaper, undried Sea Moss it did take much more to get the thickness that my customers desire and also took quite a bit more to clean. Many call this particular, sandy Sea Moss that is much thinner and takes more to clean and make into a gel, the Jamaican Sea Moss but it just hadn't been dried out and was cultivated differently, so some customers that I have sold the dried sea moss to have told me, " I don't like that Jamaican Sea Moss," when both are Jamaican Sea Moss unless he has Sea Moss from St. Lucia and I always inform my clients of which one I am selling, but remember they are both cultivated in warm waters in the Caribbean, so there really isn't a difference.

I am a business woman and have been for many years and my motto is, "the customer is always right." I love my customers and would like to stay in business, so I cater to my customers and I listen. I think of them as family, so with that being said, the customer is always right in my eyes, so we decided to stick with the drier, more expensive version of the Jamaican Sea Moss, although they do both provide the same trace minerals.

Okay. Now, back to the steps of preparing Sea Moss Gel or just Sea Moss.

Now, after you have found your vendor and are happy with the product upon receipt of the sea moss, whether it be the more sandy, thinner version or the drier, thicker version, you have now completed step one and are now onto step two, preparing the Sea Moss for consumption.

Step Two: Upon arrival and if ready to start preparing, the first thing you need to do is remove the Sea Moss from the packaging. You will then get a colander and place the sea moss into a colander and run tap water over it while massaging and removing dirt and sand. You can remove it into a bag, garbage or garbage disposal. As stated earlier, with the less drier, sandier version of Sea Moss it will take a lot of washing because it tends to be much more sandier and dirtier.

Due to the fact that this product will be consumed, you must take your time and massage and wash Sea Moss continually under running tap water, while removing dirt and sand. It usually will take you going through it anywhere from six to 10 times.

Once, you have thoroughly ran the Sea Moss under the tap water, massaged and removed the sand and dirt, six to 10 times, you will now have to soak the sea moss. I recommend using spring water. I use Zephyrhills Spring water but it's your choice.

What you will now need to do is get a bowl or a pot, whichever you prefer and get the cleaned sea moss and pour it into the bowl or pot along with the spring water of your choice and let soak for six hours to overnight. The amount of water you use should thoroughly cover the sea Moss plus two to five inches over because the sea moss is going to swell. I soak mine overnight but you can soak a minimum of four hours but I recommend at least six. You will notice that there will be a weird, distinct sea-like odor. To get rid of that odor I recommend adding a lime, split up in two pieces, that will eliminate the odor, although I do have customers that like the odor because they say they know it's authentic but that would be your preference.

Once your sea moss has soaked a minimum of 4 to six hours it is now ready for consumption or continue to be prepared as a gel.

Step Three: Now that you have received your Sea Moss, cleaned your sea moss, thoroughly soaked it in lime for four to six hours or overnight with lime, you are now ready to either continue to turn it into a gel form or eat as-is. I recommend the gel form.

Now, as previously stated you can eat it as-is in the crunchy like form or you can continue to the boiling stage to soften up and prepare for blending into a gel-form.

After allowing to soak, you will now remove the limes, if you used limes and strain out water into the colander. You will then run some more spring water into a pot for boiling. I usually put my stove's eye on medium high. You will start the stove on medium to medium high and let come to a boil, you will then place the sea moss into the pot of boiling water. It doesn't take very long for the texture to soften. It usually takes seven to ten minutes for it to soften into a more gel-like texture. Once, it softens and has boiled for the time allotted, you will then get a hand colander, which I usually get a commercial one and transfer the sea moss to a blender.

Once you transfer the sea moss to the blender, you will then blend it for approximately five to 10 seconds and it should look like a thick applesauce. If you want a thinner texture you can add a little of the boiling water but be careful or just add in some spring water from the bottle. I also have customers that put the sea moss in tea and coffee and like there's a bit thinner.

Step Four: Okay. So now you should have a gel-like texture, maybe a little thinner or a little thicker but a gel-like texture, you can now proceed to package it. You can put it in a container, I usually advise a glass container if not using jars. As a business owner, I recommend buying some canning jars and transfer the gel to the canning jars, which 16 oz. jars can be found at Wal-Mart for about \$9.00-\$11.00 for 12 jars. Once they have been packaged in the jars and caps tightened and refrigerated the gel should last you up to three months and if frozen up to six months.

Now, what I have just given you steps for is making basic, golden Sea Moss, which is our most popular version. This is the main type of sea moss that you will see on the internet in stores like Amazon, Etsy, and online stores but there are quite a few varieties and also a few recipes of many that I would like to share.

So, in our next chapter, this is what we will be discussing the different combinations, varieties, benefits when combined with other popular herbs…

No!! I did not forget….

Wild Crafted Sea Moss vs. Fake Sea Moss

Wild Crafted		Fake
Wild Crafted- Dehydrated	**Real**	**More Hydrated**
Wild Crafted – Ocean and Wild Grown	**Real**	**Taken from Pool**
Wild Crafted - Slight Sea Odor	**Real**	**Pool/Chlorine Odor**
Wild Crafted – If not dried, can be a dirty	**Real**	**Extremely dirty with salt**
Wild Crafted – thin tentacles (attach to rocks)	**Real**	**Thick tentacles**

These are some of the ways that I am able to judge the real versus the fake, but as stated previously, I only buy from one vendor and know the quality and it's guaranteed. As you continue or start your sea moss journey, you will be able to tell the difference….

Chapter Four
"Sea Moss and More"

Well, now that you have found your vendor, unpackaged your Sea Moss, cleaned your sea moss, blended into gel-form and transferred and packaged into jars, now what? Well, now you can eat it as-is or you can continue to explore different options:

Sea Moss and Elderberry:

What a beautiful combination… Yay!!!!

What is Elderberry and its benefits?

Elderberry is an edible, bluish, purple berry tree from the genus Sambucus family, having clusters of small, white flowers and small red or purplish-black berrylike fruit and is popularly used to help fight colds and flus.

One of the most popular products that we sell is Elderberry Sea Moss and Elderberry Cinnamon Sea Moss. This variation is so popular because it almost gives a double dose of vitamins. Elderberry has been used for centuries for immune support especially in the winter months and Hippocrates termed it the father of medicine. It is very high in antioxidants, Vitamin C, dietary fiber, good source of flavonols and rich in anthocyanins.

Elderberry syrup can also be purchased from a vendor or you can actually buy the berries and make the syrup yourself. If you would like to try making the Elderberry Sea Moss, I am going to recommend that you purchase the Elderberry syrup from a vendor for right now and you can usually purchase off of Etsy, Amazon or Walmart.

Elderberry Sea Moss Gel:

Follow all of the steps 1 through 4 as mentioned above but instead of packaging as the plain gold sea moss you are now going to add in one tablespoon of the elderberry, which you've purchased. So all you will need to do is still blend up the Sea Moss but just add in your tablespoon of elderberry syrup. It can be a bit bitter, depending on which vendor you purchased from, so you may need to add in in honey, agave or brown sugar and you can still can it into a canning jar and eat out of the jar or combine with other recipes.

Elderberry Sea Moss Gel with Cinnamon:

Now, the difference between our Elderberry Sea Moss Gel and our Elderberry Sea Moss Gel with Cinnamon is the Cinnamon, although when our customers order the Elderberry Sea Moss with Cinnamon they are usually doing it for a reason, Sweetness.
So with that being said, we have to sweeten it. So we do add in the teaspoon of cinnamon, ½ tsp of honey and ½ tsp of brown sugar. We do have to sometimes substitute agave in place of the honey because we have had customers that are allergic to the honey, so after reading the ingredients they do sometimes digress to the agave.

So we add in those particular products with the Sea Moss and elderberry and again pour into a canning jar and eat as-is or with tea, coffee or a smoothie. This particular product is extremely good and we have actually had a customer that overate with thyroid problems, so please do not consume no more than 2 tablespoons per day.

Extreme Nutrition, Extreme Powerhouse:

Yes, we have now addressed Sea Moss and the mineral content and we have also added in how much more powerful the sea moss is when elderberry is added but if you want to cover all 102 minerals and get total body nutrition then let me introduce you to Bladderwrack/Burdock Root and Elderberry Sea Moss.

It absolutely, without a doubt does not get any better than this.

In this blend of sea moss, elderberry, bladderwrack and burdock root, you are not only getting 92 minerals, high levels of Vitamin C and antioxidants you are now going a step further when you incorporate bladderwrack and burdock root.

What is bladderwrack and burdock root?

Bladderwrack scientifically named Fucus vesiculosus and also known by other aliases such as black tang, rock weed, sea oak, cut weed and even red fucus. This also is a sea weed and found in the North Sea, Western Baltic Sea and the Atlantic and Pacific Oceans. It also does carry a high level of iodine and was used extensively to treat goitre in 1811, which is a swelling of the thyroid gland. It is also sold as a nutritional supplement. Chemical constituents include beta-carotene, zeaxanthin, iodine, bromine, potassium and much more.

This particular sea weed is a high value mineral and is used in combination with Burdock Root.

Burdock Root is a vegetable native to Northern Asia and Europe and is also now grown in the United States. This powerhouse of antioxidants includes quercetin, luteolin and phenolic acids. It has been used for Centuries in holistic medicine to treat a variety of different conditions such as removing toxins, gastrointestinal complaints, bladder infections, syphilis, and may even inhibit certain types of cancer and cancer cell growth in another study and also treats conditions such as acne, eczema and psoriasis. It has also been used to treat colds and as a diuretic. Burdock root has also been used in a study with rats and actually had an aphrodisiac effect and did enhance sexual function on the animals.

Burdock root is packed with Vitamin B6, manganese, potassium, folate, Vitamin C, phosphorous, calcium and iron along with many other vitamins.

We do recommend to only take one teaspoon a day of this Bladderwrack/Burdock Root combination because it is packed with all 102 trace minerals that make up the body and will cover all of your daily, nutritional value that your body needs in that one teaspoon that to take more would be totally unnecessary. If you do decide to take more than one, please do not take anymore than 2 teaspoons on a daily basis.

Preparation of the Elderberry/Bladderwrack/Burdock Root Sea Moss Gel:

Once again, you will go through all of the previous steps with the original sea moss, from packaging, to cleaning, to boiling and blending. You will still then add in the elderberry in the blender with the original sea moss and you will then proceed to add-in one teaspoon of burdock root and one teaspoon of bladderwrack. You will purchase these products from your local herb store or online at your favorite herb store or Etsy. You can utilize it in its natural form or you can dry it out in powder form or purchase as powder form and add to the Sea Moss gel/elderberry mixture. These amounts of products are to be used for one 16 ounce jar of the Elderberry/Bladderwrack and Burdock Root Sea Moss Gel.

I do hope that I explained those combinations well. If I did not, please do not hesitate to reach out to me on my online store at sebiholisticgarden.com or you may also message me at sebiholisticgarden@gmail.com.

In the next chapter, Chapter 5 we will be discussing some of the benefits and or uses for Sea Moss and how to prepare and implement it into your daily lives for optimal performance in your body.

Chapter Five
"Uses and Benefits"

People use and consume sea moss in many different ways in order to reap its reward:

One way in which people consume sea moss is, of course as mentioned above, to blend it and put it into a canning jar and eat it directly out of the jar with a spoon.

One benefit that you will reap and notice almost immediately is ENERGY… OMG!!

Now, I will be honest, I can't consume a full teaspoon of sea moss daily because I am naturally energetic and I can't sleep at night. I can't even drink a half of cup of coffee at 8:00 in the morning and sleep at 10:00 at night but many of our customers actually substitute sea moss for coffee. So instead of drinking coffee, they blend it into a smoothie and drink daily or as previously mentioned, some actually blend it into their coffee or tea and drink. You really won't notice the taste. It is just a little more of a muculent like texture when added to your coffees or teas, but if you thin it out or ask whomever you purchase from to thin it out a little, then you won't notice at all.

Another benefit among many that it's known for in the Jamaican culture is for treating INFERTILITY and ERECTILE DYSFUNCTION…..

This is a big one, **HUGE**. Sea moss treatment for infertility and erectile dysfunction is a very well kept secret. Jamaican people have been consuming sea moss for many years and understands the significance of sea moss in helping women to become impregnated and stimulating sperm production in men and assisting with issues with erectile dysfunction.

I have had many customers that before purchasing has consulted with me regarding their infertility and also customers that have had issues with their husbands having a low sperm count and issues with erectile dysfunction.

As a Disclaimer, I do not proclaim to be a doctor or a scientist but I have done thorough research on my products and I do have an on-hand herbalist that has worked with and treated many patients regarding this particular issue. With that said, consuming two tablespoons of sea moss combined with a few other herbs that we sell, such as the Burdock Root and Bladderwrack, I believe (not scientifically proven) actually has assisted a few known clients with getting impregnated and has also assisted with erectile dysfunction and helped to repair damaged sperm cells and rebuild the sperm count, which in turn did lead to the woman becoming impregnated and having a baby.

I will not contribute the pregnancy fully to sea moss especially in an unscientifically based opinion, but please understand that when and/or if you do decide to consume sea moss as a dietary supplement or to assist in any ailment or body improvement, you should also commit to a lifestyle change and that should also entail a highly nutritious diet which includes a vast array of green, leafy vegetables and foods that are high in vitamins and minerals to make sure that the use of sea moss is as highly effective as possible, especially when fixing a health issue.

Although, there are soooo many uses for sea moss and I will have to write a whole nother book to go through each use there is one more that is so very important and I would like to speak briefly about.

The last use that I would like to discuss is RADIATION COMBAT.

The last few years was a surprise for everyone and caught everyone off-guard as stated earlier. I do recall many people saying that a lot of the reason why the pandemic came upon us was due to the widespread use of 5g, which in turn did prompt a large amount of sales for our business.

The reason why our sales were prompted quite abruptly due to the pandemic is because there was many conspiracy theories going around that there really wasn't a pandemic but a way for the government and internet companies to institute 5g onto our phones, that in turn means more radiation amongst us. There is such a high level of sulfur and iodine in the sea moss that it in turns helps to protect us from the radiation. The question that is then asked is, does sulfur and iodine actually protect us from radiation?

In 1945 after the bombing of Nagasaki, the director of the Department of Internal Medicine at St. Francis's Hospital fed their staff and patients not only a diet with seaweed and sea salt to combat radiation and build the immune system but also prohibited the consumption of sugar and sweets since sugar suppresses the immune system. By doing this, no one succumbed to radiation poisoning, whereas occupants and staff in other facilities that were actually farther from the blast incident that did not treat their staff accordingly did suffer from severe radiation fatalities.

Seaweeds including sea moss, which was used after the attack are very high in mineral content including the natural Iodine, which helps prevent the uptake of iodine-131, the zinc inhibits zinc-65 uptake and the sulfur is preventative for sulfur-35, which is a product of nuclear reactors. There is no foods that are more protective against radiation and environmental pollutants than sea vegetables, which has been scientifically proven.

I, honestly was not going to go into anymore direct uses for sea moss but I feel obliged to mention one more and this one is quite brief and very personal.

The last use that I must speak to you all about is SKIN AND HAIR….

Okay. Where do I start?

To use for your hair and skin you can just consume right out of the jar as previously mentioned and take orally and you will begin to see a difference in your hair and skin if taken daily and on a consistent basis.

Due to the fact that I look for a more rapid and assiduous response and because I can't consume sea moss in its recommended dosage orally on a daily basis due to the overwhelming energy that it gives me, I personally do implement the sea moss gel into my shampoo and conditioner to see a more rapid and assiduous response. So you can do both or one or the other to attain the same results. It's just that by applying directly to the skin, hair or products, you'll see a more rapid result.

Regarding the skin, I along with many customers apply the sea moss directly to the skin. I do this on a consistent basis. When applied to the skin, it is applied to the skin and allowed to set on the skin for approximately 20 minutes and rinse with cool water and pat dry with a towel.

That is one of the most unique and distinguished attributes of sea moss, it's versatility.

As you can probably tell from this book, I do have a lot to say about Sea Moss. I can honestly go on and on and on about it's uses, benefits and recipes, but I am going to save that for another book in and of itself.

Now, let's go eat.
We have decided to share a few recipes that we use on a regular basis.
Please also message me and give me your opinion on your thoughts on doing a recipe book with Sea Moss....

Chapter Six
"Recipes For You"

Spaghetti with or without meatballs:

Ingredients: Onions, green and red peppers, mushrooms, box of spaghetti pasta, 2 tablespoons of grapeseed oil, one pound of ground turkey, bag of turkey meatballs, seasoning salt, pepper, Accent, 1 tablespoon of sea moss, one jar of spaghetti sauce, Prego's Fresh Mushroom Spaghetti sauce, one tablespoon sea moss, Spaghetti noodles (your choice) and 2-3 cups of boiling water.

Cut up onions, green peppers, red peppers and mushrooms, if you wish; saute in grapeseed oil or oil of choice, stir in ground turkey and season with seasoning salt, pepper and Accent, put in approximately 1 tsp. of seasoning salt, 1 tsp of Accent and ½ tsp of black pepper, add in ¾ tablespoon of golden sea moss gel and spaghetti sauce. I personally season to taste., so the measurements above are approximations.
Also, put bag of turkey meatballs in oven for 10-15 minutes on 350 and then add in spaghetti mixture.

Right after you cut up your onions, green peppers, red peppers and mushrooms, in a separate pot start boiling the water for noodles right after sauteing the onions, greens peppers, red peppers and mushrooms are cut up and right before the ground turkey is stirred in, so that they are finished at the same time.

Allow water to come to a boil, break up spaghetti noodles in two and place in boiling water for approximately 10 minutes, after the ten minutes are up your noodles should be done. Now, get the collander again and strain the noodles into the collander and rinse with cold water. You can place them back in the pot or put in a bowl and add a little water, about a cup and pour over and a ½ tsp of oil so the noodles won't stick.   Seeing that your noodles are finished and your spaghetti sauce and turkey mixture are complete, you can eat separately by putting mixture along with meatballs on top of spaghetti noodles or mix both together.

Now, if you do decide that you want your spaghetti mixed altogether after draining the noodles, don't put any water or oil back in the pot with the noodles, just put only the noodles back in the pot and once ground turkey mixture and meatballs is finished just combine altogether and WALA, you're done.

This whole recipe will take you approximately 25-30 minutes and your sea moss is mixed in and you can't even taste or notice that it's there.

You can now serve with some pumpernickel toast and a nice salad.

Guacamole, Chips and Sour Cream (Serves 4 people):

Ingredients: Four medium sized ripe avocados, 1 tablespoon Golden Sea Moss Gel, 1/2 onion, 1 steak tomato, 1 tsp Sazon, ½ tsp black pepper, ½ tsp salt and one whole lime…

Remove skin from all four avocados
Chop up onions and tomatoes really fine
After peeling the avocados and chopping up the tomatoes and
onions, combine all ingredients together in a mixing bowl.
After all ingredients are combined together in a mixing bowl add
in your Golden Sea Moss Gel, salt, black pepper and lime
continue mixing for about five minutes or until desired textured
(some people like their guacamole chunkier and thicker and some
a bit thinner.)
You should now have your guacamole complete.
Now, it's time to get out your sour cream and blue corn chips onto
a separate plate.
You are now done and can dip your chips in the guacamole and
sour cream as desired. You can also add salsa or any other
ingredients that you may be interested in.

This again, is a great way to add sea moss gel into your routine and
get your daily minerals and not even know it's there.

This one is a great appetizer….

Green Machine Smoothie:

Ingredients: One Juicer of your choosing, One medium-sized
green apple, one stalk of celery, one leaf of kale, parsley, one
cucumber, 5" piece of ginger, 1 TSP of golden sea moss gel.

Clean and prepare your juicer for use….
Cut up green apple into approximately 6-8 pieces and remove core
(makes it easier when going into juicer.)

Cut celery into two or three pieces

Cut up Kale into two to three pieces

Get something heavy and beat the ginger down into a few pieces to make it easier to go into juicer

After cutting everything down to size, go ahead and put your sea moss gel into juicer before beginning to put the other fruits and vegetables because you'll be putting those into a shoot if you have a juicer like we have…

Basically, all you'll be doing is putting the vegetables and fruit in one at a time and it will all come out into a smoothie and your sea moss gel was put in from the initial start.

You are now ready to drink and enjoy!

This is one more way of many to consume your daily amount of sea moss and not even know that it's in there.

This particular smoothie is meant to provide you with optimal energy, nutrition and performance so it isn't catered to sweetness. If you would like it sweeter, we would recommend you add in ½ tsp peanut butter, ½ tsp honey or a half of a banana, either or all three.

These are three recipes that I recommend and that I use on a weekly basis. We have several more because sea moss can be used in just about any and everything.

We also recommend adding it to your coffees, teas, cappuccinos and other smoothies. Great way to start your day and get it out the way!!!

In Closing…..

Once again, thank you so much for your support of this book and other products. If you have any questions, concerns or comments, please do not hesitate to reach out to me or my staff.

My website is sebiholisticgarden.com or organicseamoss.shop and you can message me through our store or you may also email me directly at sebiholisticgarden@gmail.com or my Etsy store at sebiholisticgarden/etsy.com

May God and Our Ancestors Bless you and keep you.

ASE!!!